The Fit and Healthy Mediterranean Cooking Guide

Fast and Super Tasty Irresistible Recipes To Boost Your Brain

Michael Anderson

1

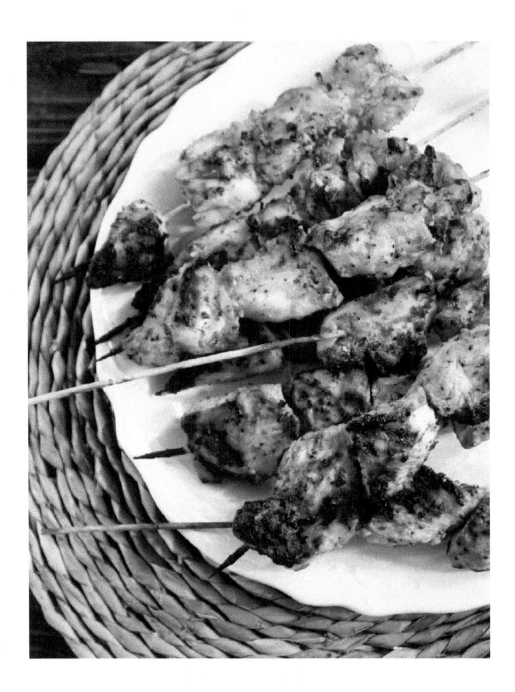

3

to date, and reliable, complete information. No warranties of any kind are declared or implied. Readers acknowledge that the author is not engaging in the rendering of legal, financial, medical or professional advice. The content within this book has been derived from various sources. Please consult a licensed professional before attempting any techniques outlined in this book.

By reading this document, the reader agrees that under no circumstances is the author responsible for any losses, direct or indirect, which are incurred as a result of the use of information contained within this document, including, but not limited to, — errors, omissions, or inaccuracies.

Table of contents

Dessert

Cardamom Almond Cream

Preparation Time: 30 minutes

Cooking Time: 0 minutes

Servings: 4

Ingredients:

- Juice of 1 lime
- 1/2 cup stevia
- 1 and 1/2 cups water
- 3 cups almond milk
- 1/2 cup honey
- 2 teaspoons cardamom, ground
- 1 teaspoon rose water
- 1 teaspoon vanilla extract

Directions:

1. In a blender, blend well the almond milk with the cardamom and the rest of the ingredients, divide into cups and keep in the fridge for 30 minutes before serving.

Nutrition:

Calories 283

Fat 11.8g

Carbohydrates 4.7g

Protein 7.1g

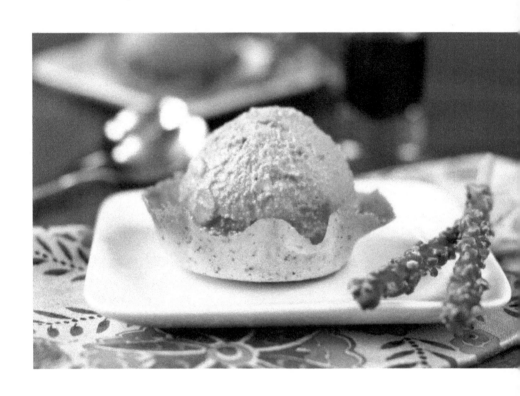

Banana Cinnamon Cupcakes

Preparation Time: 10 minutes

Cooking Time: 20 minutes

Servings: 4

Ingredients:

- 4 tablespoons avocado oil
- 4 eggs
- 1/2 cup orange juice
- 2 teaspoons cinnamon powder
- 1 teaspoon vanilla extract
- 2 bananas, peeled and chopped
- 3/4 cup almond flour
- 1/2 teaspoon baking powder
- Cooking spray

Directions:

1. In a bowl, combine the oil with the eggs, orange juice and the other ingredients except the cooking spray, whisk well, and pour in a cupcake pan greased with the cooking spray. Introduce in oven for 20 minutes, at 350 degrees F.
2. Cool the cupcakes down and serve.

Nutrition:

Calories 142; Fat 5.8g; Carbohydrates 5.7g; Protein 1.6g

Rhubarb and Apples Cream

Preparation Time: 10 minutes

Cooking Time: 0 minutes

Servings: 6

Ingredients:

- 3 cups rhubarb, chopped
- 1 and 1/2 cups stevia
- 2 eggs, whisked
- 1/2 teaspoon nutmeg, ground
- 1 tablespoon avocado oil
- 1/3 cup almond milk

Directions:

1. In a blender, combine the rhubarb with the stevia and the rest of the ingredients, pulse well, divide into cups and serve cold.

Nutrition:

Calories 20; Fat 5.2; Carbohydrates 7.6 ;Protein 2.5g

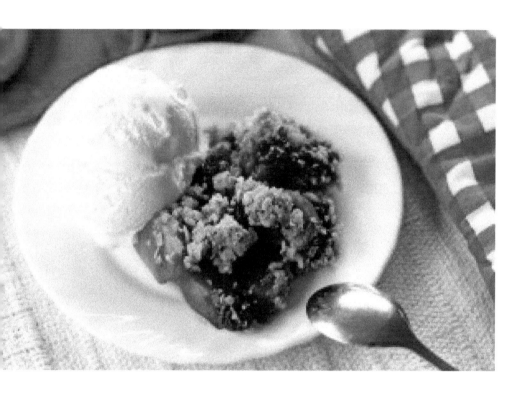

Banana Dessert with Chocolate Chips

Preparation Time: 20 minutes

Cooking Time: 30 minutes

Servings: 24

Ingredients:

- 2/3 cup white sugar
- ¾ cup butter
- 2/3 cup brown sugar
- 1 egg, beaten
- 1 tsp. vanilla extract
- 1 cup banana puree
- 1 ¾ cup flour
- 2 tsps. baking powder
- ½ tsp. salt
- 1 cup semi-sweet chocolate chips

Directions:

1. Preheat oven at 350°F. In a bowl, add the sugars and butter and beat until lightly colored. Add the egg and vanilla. Add the banana puree and stir.
2. In another bowl mix baking powder, flour, and salt. Add this mixture to the butter mixture. Stir in the chocolate chips.

16

3. Prepare a baking pan and place the dough onto it. Bake for 20 minutes and let it cool for 5 minutes before slicing into equal squares.

Nutrition:

Calories 174

Fat 8.2g

Carbs 25.2g

Protein 1.7g

Cranberry and Pistachio Biscotti

Preparation Time: 20 minutes

Cooking Time: 60 minutes

Servings: 4

Ingredients:

- ¼ cup light olive oil
- ¾ cup white sugar
- 2 tsp. vanilla extract
- ½ tsp. almond extract
- 2 eggs
- 1 ¾ cup all-purpose flour
- ¼ tsp. salt
- 1 tsp. baking powder
- ½ cup dried cranberries
- 1 ½ cup pistachio nuts

Directions:

1. Preheat the oven at 300 F. Combine olive oil and sugar in a bowl and mix well. Add eggs, almond and vanilla extracts, stir.
2. Add baking powder, salt, and flour. Add cranberries and nuts, mix. Divide the dough in half — form two 12 x 2-inch logs on a parchment baking sheet.

3. Set in the oven and bake for 35 minutes or until the blocks are golden brown. Set from oven and allow to cool for about 10 minutes.

4. Set the oven to 275 F. Cut diagonal trunks into 3/4-inch-thick slices. Place on the sides on the baking sheet covered with parchment. Bake for about 8 - 10 minutes or until dry. You can serve it both hot and cold.

Nutrition:

Calories 92

Fat 4.3g

Carbs 11.7g

Protein 2.1g

Minty Watermelon Salad

Preparation Time: 10 minutes

Cooking Time: 0 minutes

Servings: 6-8

Ingredients:

- 1 medium watermelon
- 1 cup fresh blueberries
- 2 tablespoons fresh mint leaves
- 2 tablespoons lemon juice
- 1/3 cup honey

Directions:

1. Cut the watermelon into 1-inch cubes. Put them in a bowl. Evenly distribute the blueberries over the watermelon. Chop the mint leaves and then put them into a separate bowl.
2. Add the lemon juice and honey to the mint and whisk together. Drizzle the mint dressing over the watermelon and blueberries. Serve cold.

Nutrition:

Calories 238

Fat 1g

Carbs 61g

Protein 4g

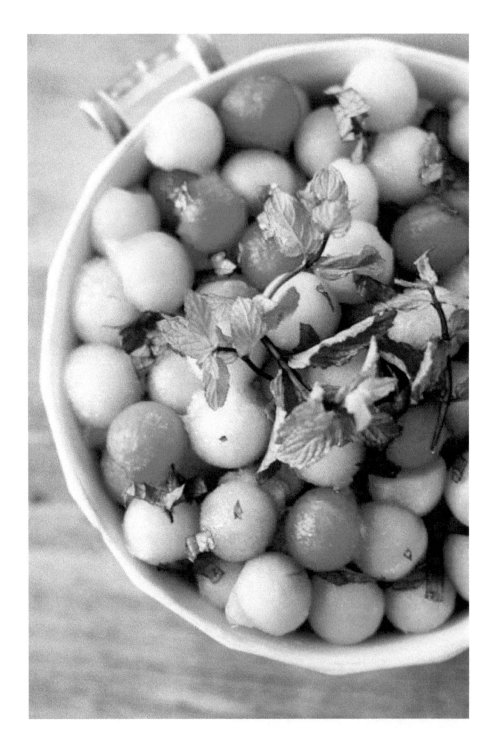

Date and Nut Balls

Preparation Time: 10 minutes

Cooking Time: 10 minutes

Servings: 6-8

Ingredients:

- 1 cup walnuts or pistachios
- 1 cup unsweetened shredded coconut
- 14 medjool dates, pits removed
- 8 tablespoons (1 stick) butter, melted

Directions:

1. Preheat the oven to 350°F. Put the nuts on a baking sheet. Toast the nuts for 5 minutes.
2. Put the shredded coconut on a clean baking sheet; toast just until it turns golden brown, about 3 to 5 minutes (coconut burns fast so keep an eye on it). Once done, remove it from the oven and put it in a shallow bowl.
3. Inside a food processor with a chopping blade, put the nuts until they have a medium chop. Put the chopped nuts into a medium bowl.
4. Add the dates and melted butter to the food processor and blend until the dates become a thick paste.

5. Pour the chopped nuts into the food processor with the dates and pulse just until the mixture is combined, about 5 to 7 pulses. Remove the mixture from the food processor and scrape it into a large bowl.

6. To make the balls, spoon 1 to 2 tablespoons of the date mixture into the palm of your hand and roll around between your hands until you form a ball. Put the ball on a clean, lined baking sheet. Repeat this until all of the mixture is formed into balls.

7. Roll each ball in the toasted coconut until the outside of the ball is coated, put the ball back on the baking sheet, and repeat.

8. Put all the balls into the fridge for 20 minutes before serving so that they firm up. You can also store any leftovers inside the fridge in an airtight container.

Nutrition:

Calories 489; Fat 35g; Carbs 48g; Protein 5g

Creamy Rice Pudding

Preparation Time: 5 minutes

Cooking Time: 45 minutes

Servings: 6

Ingredients:

- 1¼ cups long-grain rice
- 5 cups whole milk
- 1 cup sugar
- 1 tablespoon of rose water/orange blossom water
- 1 teaspoon cinnamon

Directions:

1. Rinse the rice under cold water for 30 seconds. Add the rice, milk, and sugar in a large pot. Bring to a gentle boil while continually stirring.
2. Lessen the heat to low and then let simmer for 40 to 45 minutes, stirring every 3 to 4 minutes so that the rice does not stick to the bottom of the pot.
3. Add the rose water at the end and simmer for 5 minutes. Divide the pudding into 6 bowls. Sprinkle the top with cinnamon. Let it cool for over an hour before serving. Store in the fridge.

Nutrition:

Calories 394; Fat 7g; Carbs 75g; Protein 9g

Ricotta-Lemon Cheesecake

Preparation Time: 5 minutes

Cooking Time: 1 hour

Servings: 8-10

Ingredients:

- 2 (8-ounce) packages full-fat cream cheese
- 1 (16-ounce) container full-fat ricotta cheese
- 1½ cups granulated sugar
- 1 tablespoon lemon zest
- 5 large eggs
- Nonstick cooking spray

Directions:

1. Preheat the oven to 350°F. Blend together the cream cheese and ricotta cheese. Blend in the sugar and lemon zest. Blend in the eggs; drop in 1 egg at a time, blend for 10 seconds, and repeat.
2. Put a 9-inch springform pan with a parchment paper and nonstick spray. Wrap the bottom of the pan with foil. Pour the cheesecake batter into the pan.
3. To make a water bath, get a baking or roasting pan larger than the cheesecake pan. Fill the roasting pan about 1/3 of the way up with warm water.

4. Put the cheesecake pan into the water bath. Put the whole thing in the oven and let the cheesecake bake for 1 hour.

5. After baking is complete, remove the cheesecake pan from the water bath and remove the foil. Let the cheese cake cool for 1 hour on the countertop. Then put it in the fridge to cool for at least 3 hours before serving.

Nutrition:

Calories 489

Fat 31g

Carbs 42g

Protein 15g

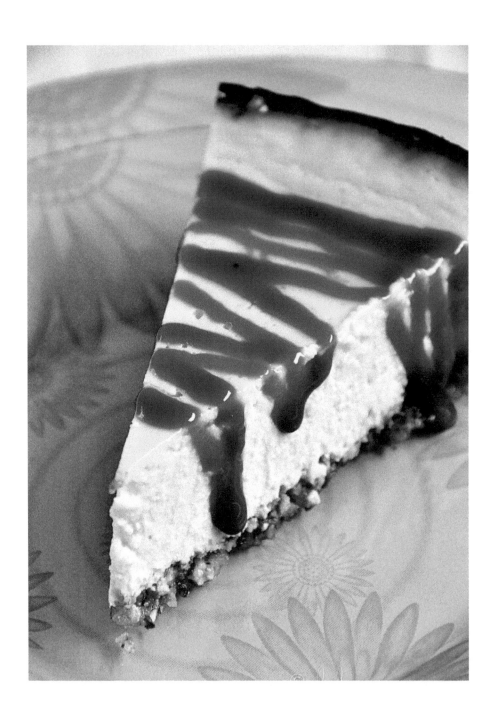

Blueberry-Blackberry Ice Pops

Preparation Time: 5 minutes + 2 hours to freeze

Cooking Time: 0 minutes

Servings: 2

Ingredients:

- ½ (13.5-ounce) can coconut cream, ¾ cup unsweetened full-fat coconut milk, or ¾ cup heavy (whipping) cream
- 2 teaspoons Swerve natural sweetener or 2 drops liquid stevia
- ½ teaspoon vanilla extract
- ¼ cup mixed blueberries and blackberries

Directions:

1. Add together the coconut cream, sweetener, and vanilla. Add the mixed berries, and then pulse just a few times. Pour it into ice pop molds and freeze for at least about 2 hours before serving.

Nutrition:

Calories: 165

Carbohydrates: 4g

Protein: 1g

Fat: 17g

Strawberry-Lime Ice Pops

Preparation Time: 5 minutes + 2 hours to freeze

Cooking Time: 0 minutes

Servings: 4

Ingredients:

½ (13.5-ounce) can coconut cream, ¾ cup unsweetened full-fat coconut milk, or ¾ cup heavy (whipping) cream

2 teaspoons Swerve natural sweetener or 2 drops liquid stevia

1 tablespoon freshly squeezed lime juice

¼ cup hulled and sliced strawberries (fresh or frozen)

Directions:

1. Mix together the coconut cream, sweetener, and lime juice in a blender. Add the strawberries, and pulse just a few times so the strawberries retain their texture.
2. Pour into ice pop molds, and freeze for at least 2 hours before serving.

Nutrition:

Calories: 166

Carbohydrates: 5g

Protein: 1g

Fat: 17g

Crockpot Keto Chocolate Cake

Preparation Time: 20 minutes

Cooking Time: 3 hours

Servings: 12

Ingredients:

- ¾ cup stevia sweetener
- 1 ½ cup almond flour
- ¼ tsp. baking powder
- ¼ cup protein powder, chocolate, or vanilla flavor
- 2/3 cup unsweetened cocoa powder
- ¼ tsp. salt
- ½ cup unsalted butter, melted
- 4 large eggs
- ¾ cup heavy cream
- 1 tsp. vanilla extract

Directions:

1. Grease the ceramic insert of the Crockpot. In a bowl, mix the sweetener, almond flour, protein powder, cocoa powder, salt, and baking powder.
2. Add the butter, eggs, cream, and vanilla extract. Pour the batter in the Crockpot and cook on low for 3 hours. Allow to cool before slicing.

Nutrition:

Calories: 253

Carbohydrates: 5.1g

Protein: 17.3g

Fat: 29.5g

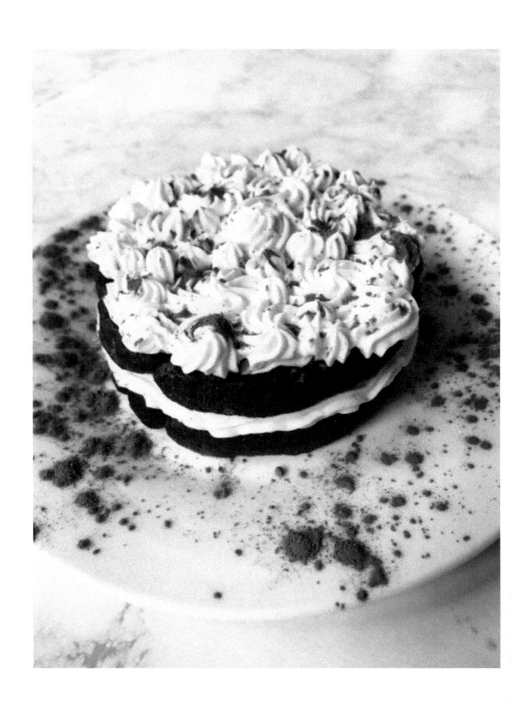

Chocolate Lava Cake

Preparation Time: 30 minutes

Cooking Time: 3 hours

Servings: 12

Ingredients:

- 1 ½ cup stevia sweetener, divided
- ½ cup almond flour
- 5 tbsps. unsweetened cocoa powder
- ½ tsp. salt
- 1 tsp. baking powder
- 3 whole eggs
- 3 egg yolks
- ½ cup butter, melted
- 1 tsp. vanilla extract
- 2 cups hot water
- 4 ounces sugar-free chocolate chips

Directions:

1. Grease the inside of the Crockpot. In a bowl, mix the stevia sweetener, almond flour, cocoa powder, salt, and baking powder.
2. In another bowl, mix the eggs, egg yolks, butter, and vanilla extract. Pour in the hot water. Pour the

wet ingredients to the dry ingredients and fold to create a batter.

3. Add the chocolate chips last. Pour into the greased Crockpot and cook on low for 3 hours. Allow to cool before serving.

Nutrition:

Calories: 157

Carbohydrates: 5.5g

Protein: 10.6g

Fat: 13g

Melomakarona

Preparation Time: 20 Minutes; **Cooking Time:** 45 Minutes

Servings: 20

Ingredients:

- 4 cups of sugar, divided
- 4 cups of water
- 1 cup plus 1 tbsp. honey, divided
- 1 (2-inch) strip orange peel, pith removed
- 1 cinnamon stick
- ½ cup extra-virgin olive oil
- ¼ cup unsalted butter,
- ¼ cup Metaxa brandy or any other brandy
- 1 tbsp. grated

Orange zest

- ¾ cup of orange juice
- ¼ tsp baking soda
- 3 cups pastry flour
- ¾ cup fine semolina flour
- 1 ½ tsp baking powder
- 4 tsp ground cinnamon, divided
- 1 tsp ground cloves, divided
- 1 cup finely chopped walnut

- 1/3 cup brown sugar

Directions:

1. Mix 3 ½ cups of sugar, 1 cup honey, orange peel, cinnamon stick, and water in a pot and heat it for about 10 minutes.

2. Mix the sugar, oil, and butter for about minutes, then add the brandy, leftover honey, and zest. Then add a mixture of baking soda and orange juice. Mix thoroughly.

3. In a distinct bowl, blend the pastry flour, baking powder, semolina, 2 tsp of cinnamon, and ½ tsp. of cloves. Add the mixture to the mixer slowly. Run the mixer until the ingredients form a dough. Cover and set aside for 30 minutes.

4. Set the oven to 350°F

5. With your palms, form small oval balls from the dough. Make a total of forty balls.

6. Bake the cookie balls for 30 minutes, then drop them in the prepared syrup.

7. Create a mixture with the walnuts, leftover cinnamon, and cloves. Spread the mixture on the top of the baked cookies. Serve the cookies and enjoy!

Nutrition:

Calories: 294kcal; Carbs: 44g; Fat: 12g; Protein: 3g

Loukoumades (Fried Honey Balls)

Preparation Time: 20 Minutes

Cooking Time: 45 Minutes

Servings: 10

Ingredients:

- 2 cups of sugar
- 1 cup of water
- 1 cup honey
- 1 ½ cups tepid water
- 1 tbsp. brown sugar
- ¼ cup of vegetable oil
- 1 tbsp. active dry yeast
- 1 ½ cups all-purpose flour, 1 cup cornstarch, ½ tsp salt
- Vegetable oil for frying
- 1 ½ cups chopped walnuts
- ¼ cup ground cinnamon

Directions:

1. Boil the sugar and water on medium heat. Add honey after 10 minutes. cool and set aside.
2. Mix the tepid water, oil, brown sugar,' and yeast in a large bowl. Allow it to sit for 10 minutes. In a

40

distinct bowl, blend the flour, salt, and cornstarch. With your hands mix the yeast and the flour to make a wet dough. Cover and set aside for 2 hours.

3. Fry in oil at 350°F. Use your palm to measure the sizes of the dough as they are dropped in the frying pan. Fry each batch for about 3-4 minutes.

4. Immediately the loukoumades are done frying, drop them in the prepared syrup.

5. Serve with cinnamon and walnuts.

Nutrition:

Calories: 355kcal

Carbs: 64g

Fat: 7g

Protein: 6g

Cocoa Brownies

Preparation Time: 10 minutes

Cooking Time: 20 minutes

Servings: 8

Ingredients:

- 30 ounces canned lentils, rinsed and drained
- 1 tablespoon honey
- 1 banana, peeled and chopped
- 1/2 teaspoon baking soda
- 4 tablespoons almond butter
- 2 tablespoons cocoa powder
- Cooking spray

Directions:

1. In a food processor, pulse well the lentils with the honey and the other ingredients except the cooking spray.
2. Transfer this into a pan greased with cooking spray, lay evenly, introduce in the oven at 375 degrees F for 20 minutes. Slice the brownies and serve cold.

Nutrition:

Calories 200; Fat 4.5g; Carbohydrates 8.7g; Protein4.3g

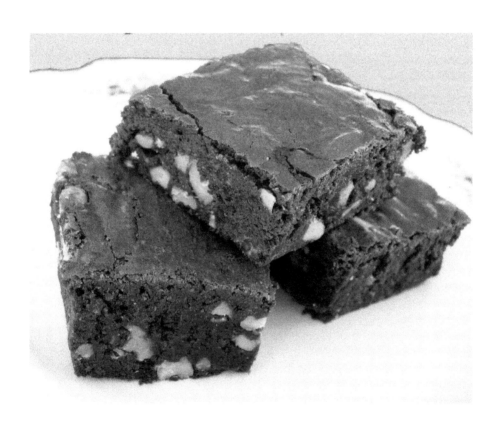

Breakfast

Low-Carb Baked Eggs with Avocado and Feta

Preparation Time: 10 minutes

Cooking Time: 15 minutes

Servings: 2

Ingredients:

- 1 avocado
- 4 eggs
- 2-3 tbsp. crumbled feta cheese
- Nonstick cooking spray
- Pepper and salt to taste

Directions:

1. First, you will have to preheat the oven to 400 degrees F. After that, when the oven is on the proper temperature, you will have to put the gratin dishes right on the baking sheet.

2. Then, leave the dishes to heat in the oven for almost 10 minutes After that process, you need to break the eggs into individual ramekins.

3. Then, let the avocado and eggs come to room temperature for at least 10 minutes. Then, peel the avocado properly and cut it each half into 6-8 slices.

4. You will have to remove the dishes from the oven and spray them with the non-stick spray. Then, you will have to arrange all the sliced avocados in the dishes and tip two eggs into each dish. Sprinkle with feta, add pepper and salt to taste, serve.

Nutrition:

Calories: 280

Protein: 11 g

Fat: 23 g

Carbs: 10 g

Mediterranean Eggs White Breakfast Sandwich with Roasted Tomatoes

 Preparation Time: 15 minutes

Cooking Time: 10 minutes

Servings: 2

Ingredients:

- Salt and pepper to taste
- ¼ cup egg whites
- 1 teaspoon chopped fresh herbs like rosemary, basil, parsley,
- 1 whole-grain seeded ciabatta roll
- 1 teaspoon butter
- 1-2 slices Muenster cheese
- 1 tablespoon pesto
- About ½ cup roasted tomatoes
- 10 ounces grape tomatoes
- 1 tablespoon extra-virgin olive oil
- Black pepper and salt to taste

Directions:

1. First, you will have to melt the butter over medium heat in the small nonstick skillet. Then, mix the egg whites with pepper and salt.

48

2. Then, sprinkle it with the fresh herbs. After that cook it for almost 3-4 minutes or until the eggs are done, then flip it carefully.
3. Meanwhile, toast ciabatta bread in the toaster. Place the egg on the bottom half of the sandwich rolls, then top with cheese
4. Add roasted tomatoes and the top half of roll. To make a roasted tomato, preheat the oven to 400 degrees. Then, slice the tomatoes in half lengthwise.
5. Place on the baking sheet and drizzle with olive oil. Season it with pepper and salt and then roast in the oven for about 20 minutes. Skins will appear wrinkled when done.

Nutrition:

Calories: 458, Protein: 21 g, Fat: 24 g, Carbs: 51 g

Greek Yogurt Pancakes

Preparation Time: 10 minutes

Cooking Time: 5 minutes

Servings: 2

Ingredients:

- 1 cup all-purpose flour
- 1 cup whole-wheat flour
- 1/4 teaspoon salt
- 4 teaspoons baking powder
- 1 tablespoon sugar
- 1 1/2 cups unsweetened almond milk
- 2 teaspoons vanilla extract
- 2 large eggs
- 1/2 cup plain 2% Greek yogurt
- Fruit, for serving
- Maple syrup, for serving

Directions:

1. First, you will have to pour the curds into the bowl and mix them well until creamy. After that, you will have to add egg whites and mix them well until combined.

2. Then take a separate bowl, pour the wet mixture into the dry mixture. Stir to combine. The batter will be extremely thick.

3. Then, simply spoon the batter onto the sprayed pan heated too medium-high. The batter must make 4 large pancakes.

4. Then, you will have to flip the pancakes once when they start to bubble a bit on the surface. Cook until golden brown on both sides.

Nutrition:

Calories: 166

Protein: 14 g

Fat: 5 g

Carbs: 52g

Mediterranean Feta and Quinoa Egg Muffins

Preparation Time: 15 minutes

Cooking Time: 15 minutes

Servings: 12

Ingredients:

- 2 cups baby spinach finely chopped
- 1 cup chopped or sliced cherry tomatoes
- 1/2 cup finely chopped onion
- 1 tablespoon chopped fresh oregano
- 1 cup crumbled feta cheese
- 1/2 cup chopped {pitted} kalamata olives
- 2 teaspoons high oleic sunflower oil
- 1 cup cooked quinoa
- 8 eggs
- 1/4 teaspoon salt

Directions:

1. Pre-heat oven to 350 degrees Fahrenheit, and then prepare 12 silicone muffin holders on the baking sheet, or just grease a 12-cup muffin tin with oil and set aside.

2. Finely chop the vegetables and then heat the skillet to medium. After that, add the vegetable oil and onions and sauté for 2 minutes.
3. Then, add tomatoes and sauté for another minute, then add spinach and sauté until wilted, about 1 minute.
4. Place the beaten egg into a bowl and then add lots of vegetables like feta cheese, quinoa, veggie mixture as well as salt, and then stir well until everything is properly combined.
5. Pour the ready mixture into greased muffin tins or silicone cups, dividing the mixture equally. Then, bake it in an oven for 30 minutes or so.

Nutrition:

Calories: 113, Protein: 6 g, Fat: 7 g, Carbs: 5 g

Mediterranean Eggs

Preparation Time: 15 minutes

Cooking Time: 20 minutes

Servings: 2

Ingredients:

- 5 tbsp. of divided olive oil
- 2 diced medium-sized Spanish onions
- 2 diced red bell peppers
- 2 minced cloves garlic
- 1 teaspoon cumin seeds
- 4 diced large ripe tomatoes
- 1 tablespoon of honey
- Salt
- Freshly ground black pepper
- 1/3 cup crumbled feta
- 4 eggs
- 1 teaspoon zaatar spice
- Grilled pita during serving

Directions:

1. Add 3 tablespoons of olive oil into a pan and heat it over medium heat. Along with the oil, sauté the cumin seeds, onions, garlic, and red pepper for a few minutes.

54

2. After that, add the diced tomatoes and salt and pepper to taste and cook them for about 10 minutes till they come together and form a light sauce.
3. With that, half the preparation is already done. Now you just have to break the eggs directly into the sauce and poach them.
4. However, you must keep in mind to cook the egg whites but keep the yolks still runny. This takes about 8 to 10 minutes.
5. While plating adds some feta and olive oil with zaatar spice to further enhance the flavors. Once done, serve with grilled pita.

Nutrition:

Calories: 304, Protein: 12 g, Fat: 16 g, Carbs: 28 g

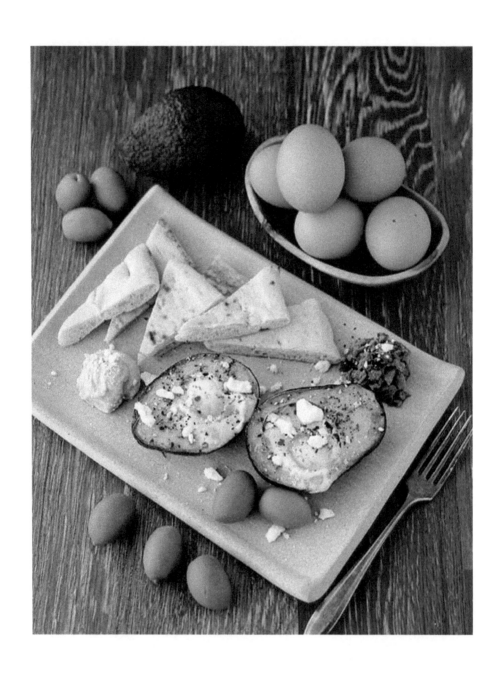

Pastry-Less Spanakopita

Preparation Time: 5 minutes

Cooking Time: 20 minutes

Servings: 4

Ingredients:

- 1/8 teaspoons black pepper, add as per taste
- 1/3 cup of Extra virgin olive oil
- 4 lightly beaten eggs
- 7 cups of Lettuce, preferably a spring mix (mesclun)
- 1/2 cup of crumbled Feta cheese
- 1/8 teaspoon of Sea salt, add to taste
- 1 finely chopped medium Yellow onion

Directions:

1. Warm the oven to 180C and grease the flan dish. Once done, pour the extra virgin olive oil into a large saucepan and heat it over medium heat with the onions, until they are translucent.

2. Add greens and keep stirring until all the ingredients are wilted. Season it with salt and pepper and transfer the greens to the prepared dish and sprinkle on some feta cheese.

3. Pour the eggs and bake it for 20 minutes till it is cooked through and slightly brown.

Nutrition:

Calories: 325

Protein: 11.2 g

Fat: 27.9 g

Carbs: 7.3 g

Date and Walnut Overnight Oats

Preparation Time: 5 minutes

Cooking Time: 20 minutes

Servings: 2

Ingredients:

- ¼ Cup Greek Yogurt, Plain
- 1/3 cup of yogurt
- 2/3 cup of oats
- 1 cup of milk
- 2 tsp date syrup or you can also use maple syrup or honey
- 1 mashed banana
- ¼ tsp cinnamon
- ¼ cup walnuts
- pinch of salt (approx.1/8 tsp)

Directions:

1. Firstly, get a mason jar or a small bowl and add all the ingredients. After that stir and mix all the ingredients well. Cover it securely, and cool it in a refrigerator overnight.
2. After that, take it out the next morning, add more liquid or cinnamon if required, and serve cold.

(However, you can also microwave it for people with a warmer palate.)

Nutrition:

Calories: 350

Protein: 14 g

Fat: 12 g

Carbs: 49 g

Lunch

Curry and Lime Green Beans

Preparation Time: 10 minutes

Cooking Time: 25 minutes

Servings: 4

Ingredients:

- 2 tablespoons olive oil
- 1 yellow onion, chopped
- 1 pound green beans, trimmed
- 2 teaspoons garlic, minced
- A pinch of salt and black pepper
- 2 teaspoons curry powder
- 1/2 cup vegetable stock
- 1/2 teaspoon brown mustard seeds
- 1 tablespoon lime juice

Directions:

1. Heat up a large pan with the oil over medium-high heat, add the onion and the garlic and sauté for 5 minutes.
2. Add the green beans and the other ingredients, toss, cook over medium heat for 20 minutes, divide between plates and serve.

Nutrition:

Calories 181

Fat 3

Fiber 6

Carbs 12

Protein 6

Mediterranean Cod Stew

Prep time: 10 minutes | Cook time: 20 minutes | Serves 6

2 tablespoons extra-virgin olive oil

2 cups chopped onion

2 garlic cloves, minced

¾ teaspoon smoked paprika

1 (14.5-ounce / 411-g) can diced tomatoes, undrained

1 (12-ounce / 340-g) jar roasted red peppers, drained and chopped

1 cup sliced olives, green or black

1⅓ cup dry red wine

¼ teaspoon kosher or sea salt

¼ teaspoon freshly ground black pepper

1½ pounds (680 g) cod fillets, cut into 1-inch pieces

3 cups sliced mushrooms

1. In a large stockpot over medium heat, heat the oil. Add the onion and cook for 4 minutes, stirring occasionally. Add the garlic and smoked paprika and cook for 1 minute, stirring often.

2. Mix in the tomatoes with their juices, roasted peppers, olives, wine, pepper, and salt, and turn the heat to medium-high. Bring the

mixture to a boil. Add the cod fillets and mushrooms, and reduce the heat to medium.

3. Cover and cook for about 10 minutes, stirring a few times, until the cod is cooked through and flakes easily, and serve.

Per Serving

calories: 167 | fat: 5.0g | protein: 19.0g | carbs: 11.0g | fiber: 5.0g | sodium: 846mg

Chili Avocado and Onion Salad

Preparation Time: 10 minutes

Cooking Time: 0 minutes

Servings: 4

Ingredients:

- 2 red onions, sliced
- 2 avocados, peeled, pitted and roughly sliced
- 1 tablespoon olive oil
- 1 tablespoon balsamic vinegar
- 1 tablespoon dill, chopped
- 1 teaspoon chili powder
- A pinch of salt and black pepper

Directions:

1. In a bowl, pour the avocado with the onions and the other ingredients, toss, and serve.

Nutrition:

Calories 171

Fat 2

Fiber 7

Carbs 13

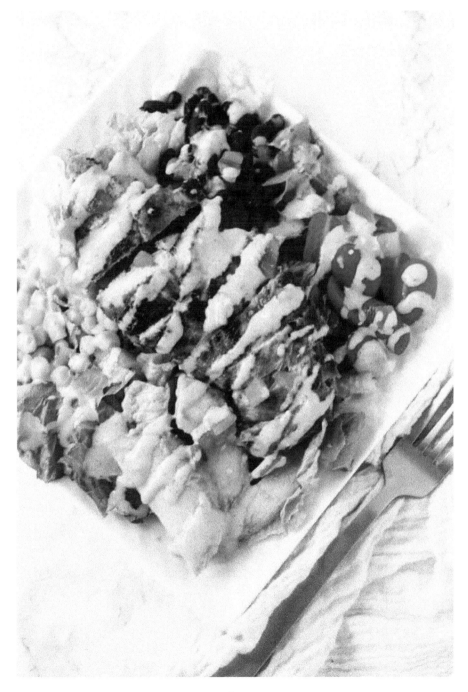

Hot Green Beans

Preparation Time: 10 minutes

Cooking Time: 20 minutes

Servings: 4

Ingredients:

- 1 pound green beans, trimmed and halved
- 1 cup radishes, sliced
- 2 tablespoons olive oil
- 1 yellow onion, chopped
- A pinch of salt and black pepper
- 4 scallions, chopped
- 1 teaspoon chili flakes
- 1 tablespoon cilantro,

Directions:

1. Heat up the pan with oil, add the onion and the scallions and sauté for 5 minutes.
2. Add the green beans and the other ingredients, toss, cook over medium heat for 15 minutes, divide between plates and serve.

Nutrition:

Calories 60

Fat 3

Fiber 2

Carbs 5

Protein 1

Halibut and Quinoa Mix

Preparation Time: 10 minutes

Cooking Time: 12 minutes

Servings: 4

Ingredients:

- 4 halibut fillets, boneless
- 2 tablespoons olive oil
- 1 teaspoon rosemary, dried
- 2 teaspoons cumin, ground
- 1 tablespoons coriander, ground
- 2 teaspoons cinnamon powder
- 2 teaspoons oregano, dried
- A pinch of salt and black pepper
- 2 cups quinoa, cooked
- 1 cup cherry tomatoes, halved
- 1 avocado, peeled, pitted and sliced
- 1 cucumber, cubed
- 1/2 cup black olives
- Juice of 1 lemon

Directions:

1. In a bowl, combine the fish with the rosemary, cumin, coriander, cinnamon, oregano, salt and pepper and toss.

2. Heat up the pan with oil adds the fish, and sear for 2 minutes on each side.
3. Introduce the pan in the oven and bake the fish at 425 degrees F for 7 minutes.
4. Meanwhile, in a bowl, mix the quinoa with the remaining ingredients, toss and divide between plates.
5. Add the fish next to the quinoa mix and serve right away.

Nutrition:

Calories 364, Fat 15.4, Fiber 11.2, Carbs 56.4, Protein 24.5

Lemon and Dates Barramundi

Preparation Time: 10 minutes

Cooking Time: 12 minutes

Servings: 2

Ingredients:

- 2 barramundi fillets, boneless
- 1 shallot, sliced
- 4 lemon slices
- Juice of 1/2 lemon
- Zest of 1 lemon, grated
- 2 tablespoons olive oil
- 6 ounces baby spinach
- 1/4 cup almonds, chopped
- 4 dates, pitted and chopped
- 1/4 cup parsley, chopped
- Salt and black pepper to the taste

Directions:

1. Flavor the fish with salt and pepper and arrange on 2 parchment paper pieces.
2. Top the fish with the lemon slices, drizzle the lemon juice, and then top with the other ingredients except the oil.

3. Drizzle 1 tablespoon oil over each fish mix, wrap the parchment paper around the fish shaping to packets and arrange them on a baking sheet.
4. Bake at 400 degrees F for 12 minutes, cool the mix a bit, unfold, divide everything between plates and serve.

Nutrition:

Calories 232,

Fat 16.5,

Fiber 11.1,

Carbs 24.8,

Protein 6.5

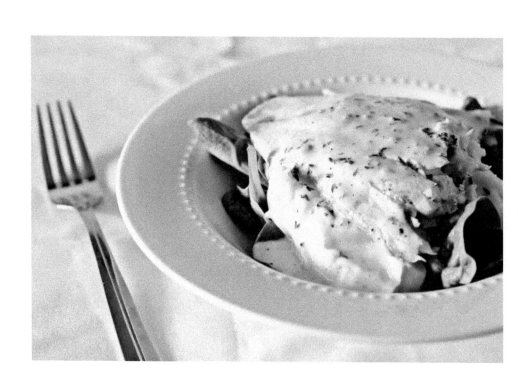

Fish Cakes

Preparation Time: 10 minutes

Cooking Time: 10 minutes

Servings: 6

Ingredients:

- 20 ounces canned sardines, drained and mashed well
- 2 garlic cloves, minced
- 2 tablespoons dill, chopped
- 1 yellow onion, chopped
- 1 cup panko breadcrumbs
- 1 egg, whisked
- A pinch of salt and black pepper
- 2 tablespoons lemon juice
- 5 tablespoons olive oil

Directions:

1. In a bowl, combine the sardines with the garlic, dill and the rest of the ingredients except the oil, stir well and shape medium cakes out of this mix.
2. Heat up the pan with oil, add the fish cakes, and cook for 5 minutes on each side.
3. Serve the cakes with a side salad.

Nutrition:

Calories 288,

Fat 12.8,

Fiber 10.2,

Carbs 22.2,

Protein 6.8

Catfish Fillets and Rice

Preparation Time: 10 minutes

Cooking Time: 55 minutes

Servings: 2

Ingredients:

- 2 catfish fillets, boneless
- 2 tablespoons Italian seasoning
- 2 tablespoons olive oil
- For the rice:
- 1 cup brown rice
- 2 tablespoons olive oil
- 1 and 1/2 cups water
- 1/2 cup green bell pepper, chopped
- 2 garlic cloves, minced
- 1/2 cup white onion, chopped
- 2 teaspoons Cajun seasoning
- 1/2 teaspoon garlic powder
- Salt and black pepper to the taste

Directions:

1. Heat up a pot with 2 tablespoons oil over medium heat, add the onion, garlic, garlic powder, salt and pepper and sauté for 5 minutes.

2. Add the rice, water, bell pepper and the seasoning, bring to a simmer and cook over medium heat for 40 minutes.
3. Heat up the pan with oil, add the fish and the Italian seasoning, and cook for 5 minutes on each side.
4. Divide the rice between plates, add the fish on top and serve.

Nutrition:

Calories 261,

Fat 17.6,

Fiber 12.2,

Carbs 24.8,

Protein 12.5

Halibut Pan

Preparation Time: 10 minutes

Cooking Time: 20 minutes

Servings: 4

Ingredients:

- 4 halibut fillets, boneless
- 1 red bell pepper, chopped
- 2 tablespoons olive oil
- 1 yellow onion, chopped
- 4 garlic cloves, minced
- 1/2 cup chicken stock
- 1 teaspoon basil, dried
- 1/2 cup cherry tomatoes, halved
- 1/3 cup calamite olives
- Salt and black pepper to the taste

Directions:

1. Heat up a pan with the oil over medium heat, add the fish, cook for 5 minutes on each side and divide between plates.
2. Add the onion, bell pepper, garlic and tomatoes to the pan, stir and sauté for 3 minutes.

3. Add salt, pepper and the rest of the ingredients, toss, cook for 3 minutes more, divide next to the fish and serve.

Nutrition:

Calories 253,

Fat 8,

Fiber 1,

Carbs 5,

Protein 28

Baked Shrimp Mix

Preparation Time: 10 minutes

Cooking Time: 32 minutes

Servings: 4

Ingredients:

- 4 gold potatoes, peeled and sliced
- 2 fennel bulbs
- 2 shallots, chopped
- 2 garlic cloves, minced
- 3 tablespoons olive oil
- 1/2 cup calamite olives
- 2 pounds shrimp, peeled and deveined
- 1 teaspoon lemon zest, grated
- 2 teaspoons oregano, dried
- 4 ounces feta cheese, crumbled
- 2 tablespoons parsley, chopped

Directions:

1. In a roasting pan, combine the potatoes with 2 tablespoons oil, garlic and the rest of the ingredients except the shrimp, toss, introduce in the oven and bake at 450 degrees F for 25 minutes.
2. Add the shrimp, toss, bake for 7 minutes more, divide between plates and serve.

Nutrition:

Calories 341,

Fat 19,

Fiber 9,

Carbs 34,

Protein 10

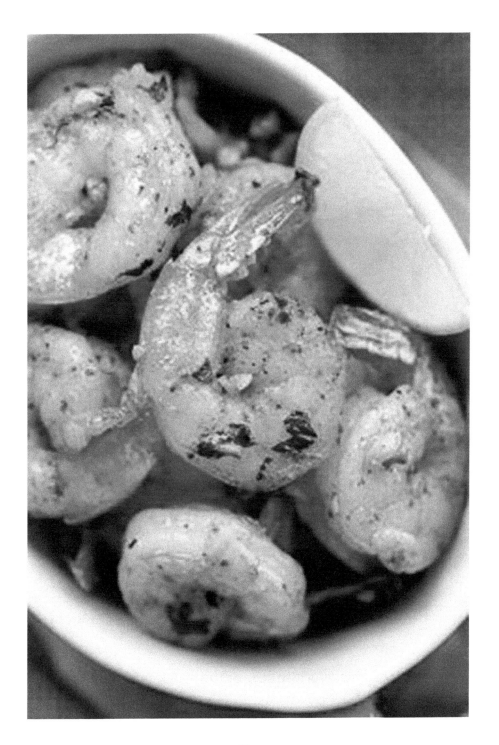

Shrimp and Lemon Sauce

Preparation Time: 10 minutes

Cooking Time: 15 minutes

Servings: 4

Ingredients:

- 1 pound shrimp, peeled and deveined
- 1/3 cup lemon juice
- 4 egg yolks
- 2 tablespoons olive oil
- 1 cup chicken stock
- Salt and black pepper to the taste
- 1 cup black olives, pitted and halved
- 1 tablespoon thyme, chopped

Directions:

1. In a bowl, merge the lemon juice with the egg yolks and whisk well.
2. Heat up the pan with oil, add the shrimp and cook for 2 and transfer to a plate.
3. Heat up a pan with the stock over medium heat, add some of this over the egg yolks and lemon juice mix and whisk well.
4. Add this over the rest of the stock, also add salt and pepper, whisk well and simmer for 2 minutes.

5. Attach the shrimp and the rest of the ingredients, toss and serve right away.

Nutrition:

Calories 237,

Fat 15.3,

Fiber 4.6,

Carbs 15.4,

Protein 7.6

Shrimp and Beans Salad

Preparation Time: 10 minutes

Cooking Time: 4 minutes

Servings: 4

Ingredients:

- 1 pound shrimp, peeled and deveined
- 30 ounces canned cannellini beans
- 2 tablespoons olive oil
- 1 cup cherry tomatoes, halved
- 1 teaspoon lemon zest, grated
- 1/2 cup red onion, chopped
- 4 handfuls baby arugula
- A pinch of salt and black pepper
- For the dressing:
- 3 tablespoons red wine vinegar
- 2 garlic cloves, minced
- 1/2 cup olive oil

Directions:

1. Heat up the pan with oil, add the shrimp and cook for 2 minutes on each side.
2. In a salad bowl, combine the shrimp with the beans and the rest of the ingredients except the ones for the dressing and toss.

3. In a separate bowl, combine the vinegar with 1/2 cup oil and the garlic and whisk well.

4. Pour over the salad, toss and serve right away.

Nutrition:

Calories 207,

Fat 12.3,

Fiber 6.6,

Carbs 15.4,

Protein 8.7

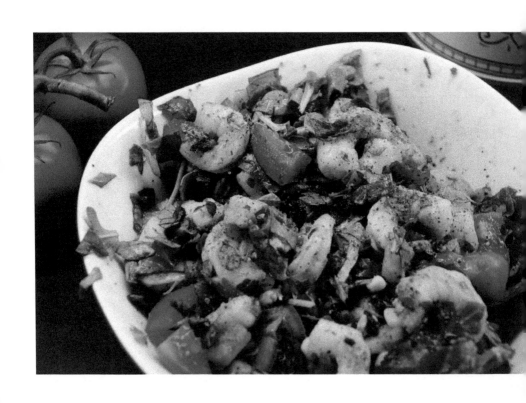

Creamy Chicken Breasts

Preparation Time: 10 minutes

Cooking Time: 12 minutes

Servings: 4

Ingredients:

- 4 chicken breasts, skinless and boneless
- 1 tbsp basil pesto
- 1 1/2 tbsp cornstarch
- 1/4 cup roasted red peppers, chopped
- 1/3 cup heavy cream
- 1 tsp Italian seasoning
- 1 tsp garlic, minced
- 1 cup chicken broth
- Pepper
- Salt

Directions:

1. Add chicken into the Pressure Pot. Season chicken with Italian seasoning, pepper, and salt. Sprinkle with garlic. Pour broth over chicken. Seal pot with lid and cook on high for 8 minutes.
2. Once done, allow to release pressure naturally for 5 minutes then release remaining using quick release.

Remove lid. Transfer chicken on a plate and clean the Pressure Pot.

3. Set Pressure Pot on sauté mode. Add heavy cream, pesto, cornstarch, and red pepper to the pot and stir well and cook for 3-4 minutes.
4. Return chicken to the pot and coat well with the sauce. Serve and enjoy.

Nutrition:

Calories 341

Fat 15.2 g

Carbohydrates 4.4 g

Protein 43.8 g

Cheese Garlic Chicken & Potatoes

Preparation Time: 10 minutes

Cooking Time: 13 minutes

Servings: 4

Ingredients:

- 2 lb. chicken breasts, skinless, boneless, cut into chunks
- 1 tbsp olive oil
- 3/4 cup chicken broth
- 1 tbsp Italian seasoning
- 1 tbsp garlic powder
- 1 tsp garlic, minced
- 1 1/2 cup parmesan cheese, shredded
- 1 lb. potatoes, chopped
- Pepper
- Salt

Directions:

1. Add oil into the inner pot of Pressure Pot and set the pot on sauté mode. Add chicken and cook until browned. Add remaining ingredients except for cheese and stir well.
2. Seal pot with lid and cook on high for 8 minutes. Once done, release pressure using quick release.

91

Remove lid. Top with cheese and cover with lid for 5 minutes or until cheese is melted. Serve and enjoy.

Nutrition:

Calories 674

Fat 29 g

Carbohydrates 21.4 g

Protein 79.7 g

Easy Chicken Scampi

Preparation Time: 10 minutes

Cooking Time: 25 minutes

Servings: 4

Ingredients:

- 3 chicken breasts, skinless, boneless, and sliced
- 1 tsp garlic, minced
- 1 tbsp Italian seasoning
- 2 cups chicken broth
- 1 bell pepper, sliced
- 1/2 onion, sliced
- Pepper
- Salt

Directions:

1. Add chicken into the Pressure Pot and top with remaining ingredients. Seal pot with lid and cook on high for 25 minutes. Once done, release pressure using quick release. Remove lid.
2. Remove chicken from pot and shred using a fork. Return shredded chicken to the pot and stir well. Serve over cooked whole grain pasta and top with cheese.

Nutrition:

Calories 254; Fat 9.9 g; Carbohydrates 4.6 g; Protein 34.6 g

Protein Packed Chicken Bean Rice

Preparation Time: 10 minutes

Cooking Time: 15 minutes

Servings: 6

Ingredients:

- 1 lb. chicken breasts, skinless, boneless, and cut into chunks
- 14 oz can cannellini beans, rinsed and drained
- 4 cups chicken broth
- 2 cups brown rice
- 1 tbsp Italian seasoning
- 1 small onion, chopped
- 1 tbsp garlic, chopped
- 1 tbsp olive oil
- Pepper
- Salt

Directions:

1. Add oil into the inner pot of Pressure Pot and set the pot on sauté mode. Add garlic and onion and sauté for 3 minutes. Add remaining ingredients and stir everything well.

2. Seal pot with a lid and select manual and set timer for 12 minutes. Once done, release pressure using quick release. Remove lid. Stir well and serve.

Nutrition:

Calories 494; Fat 11.3 g; Carbohydrates 61.4 g; Protein 34.2 g

Pesto Vegetable Chicken

Preparation Time: 10 minutes

Cooking Time: 25 minutes

Servings: 4

Ingredients:

- 1 1/2 lb. chicken thighs, skinless, boneless, and cut into pieces
- 1/2 cup chicken broth
- 1/4 cup fresh parsley, chopped
- 2 cups cherry tomatoes, halved
- 1 cup basil pesto
- 3/4 lb. asparagus, trimmed and cut in half
- 2/3 cup sun-dried tomatoes, drained and chopped
- 2 tbsp olive oil
- Pepper
- Salt

Directions:

1. Add oil into the inner pot of Pressure Pot and set the pot on sauté mode. Add chicken and sauté for 5 minutes. Add remaining ingredients except for tomatoes and stir well.

2. Seal pot with a lid and select manual and set timer for 15 minutes. Once done, release pressure using quick release. Remove lid.
3. Add tomatoes and stir well. Again, seal the pot and select manual and set timer for 5 minutes. Release pressure using quick release. Remove lid. Stir well and serve.

Nutrition:

Calories 459

Fat 20.5 g

Carbohydrates 14.9 g

Protein 9.2 g

Greek Chicken Rice

Preparation Time: 10 minutes

Cooking Time: 14 minutes

Servings: 4

Ingredients:

- 3 chicken breasts, skinless, boneless, and cut into chunks
- ¼ fresh parsley, chopped
- 1 zucchini, sliced
- 2 bell peppers, chopped
- 1 cup rice, rinsed and drained
- 1 ½ cup chicken broth
- 1 tbsp oregano
- 3 tbsp fresh lemon juice
- 1 tbsp garlic, minced
- 1 onion, diced
- 2 tbsp olive oil
- Pepper
- Salt

Directions:

1. Add oil into the inner pot of Pressure Pot and set the pot on sauté mode. Add onion and chicken and cook for 5 minutes. Add rice, oregano, lemon juice,

99

garlic, broth, pepper, and salt and stir everything well.

2. Seal pot with lid and cook on high for 4 minutes. Once done, release pressure using quick release. Remove lid. Add parsley, zucchini, and bell peppers and stir well.

3. Seal pot again with lid and select manual and set timer for 5 minutes. Release pressure using quick release. Remove lid. Stir well and serve.

Nutrition:

Calories 500

Fat 16.5 g

Carbohydrates 48 g

Protein 38.7 g

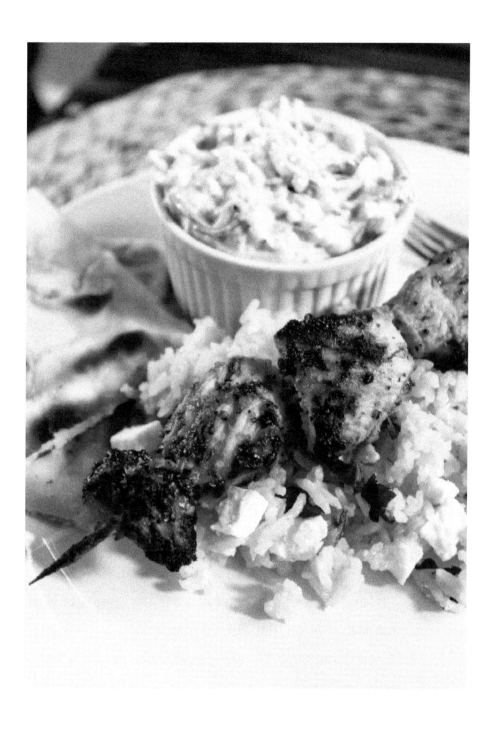

Flavorful Chicken Tacos

Preparation Time: 10 minutes

Cooking Time: 10 minutes

Servings: 3

Ingredients:

- 2 chicken breasts, skinless and boneless
- 1 tbsp chili powder
- 1/2 tsp ground cumin
- 1/2 tsp garlic powder
- 1/4 tsp onion powder
- 1/2 tsp paprika
- 4 oz can green chilis, diced
- 1/4 cup chicken broth
- 14 oz can tomato, diced
- Pepper
- Salt

Directions:

1. Add all ingredients except chicken into the Pressure Pot and stir well. Add chicken and stir. Seal pot with lid and cook on high for 10 minutes.
2. Once done, allow to release pressure naturally for 5 minutes then release remaining using quick release. Remove lid.

3. Remove chicken from pot and shred using a fork. Return shredded chicken to the pot and stir well. Serve and enjoy.

Nutrition:

Calories 237

Fat 8 g

Carbohydrates 10.8 g

Protein 30.5 g

Quinoa Chicken Bowls

Preparation Time: 10 minutes

Cooking Time: 6 minutes

Servings: 4

Ingredients:

- 1 lb. chicken breasts, skinless, boneless, and cut into chunks
- 14 oz can chickpeas, drained and rinsed
- 1 cup olives, pitted and sliced
- 1 cup cherry tomatoes, halved
- 1 cucumber, sliced
- 2 tsp Greek seasoning
- 1 1/2 cups chicken broth
- 1 cup quinoa, rinsed and drained
- Pepper
- Salt

Directions:

1. Add broth and quinoa into the Pressure Pot and stir well. Season chicken with Greek seasoning, pepper, and salt and place into the Pressure Pot.
2. Seal pot with lid and cook on high for 6 minutes. Once done, release pressure using quick release. Remove lid. Stir quinoa and chicken mixture well.

3. Add remaining ingredients and stir everything well. Serve immediately and enjoy it.

Nutrition:

Calories 566

Fat 16.4 g

Carbohydrates 57.4 g

Protein 46.8 g

Quick Chicken with Mushrooms

Preparation Time: 10 minutes

Cooking Time: 22 minutes

Servings: 6

Ingredients:

- 2 lb. chicken breasts, skinless and boneless
- 1/2 cup heavy cream
- 1/3 cup water
- 3/4 lb. mushrooms, sliced
- 3 tbsp olive oil
- 1 tsp Italian seasoning
- Pepper
- Salt

Directions:

1. Add oil into the inner pot of Pressure Pot and set the pot on sauté mode. Season chicken with Italian seasoning, pepper, and salt.
2. Add chicken to the pot and sauté for 5 minutes. Remove chicken from pot and set aside. Add mushrooms and sauté for 5 minutes or until mushrooms are lightly brown.

3. Return chicken to the pot. Add water and stir well. Seal pot with a lid and select manual and set timer for 12 minutes.
4. Once done, release pressure using quick release. Remove lid. Remove chicken from pot and place on a plate.
5. Set pot on sauté mode. Add heavy cream and stir well and cook for 5 minutes. Pour mushroom sauce over chicken and serve.

Nutrition:

Calories 396

Fat 22.3 g

Carbohydrates 2.2 g

Protein 45.7 g

Herb Garlic Chicken

Preparation Time: 10 minutes

Cooking Time: 12 minutes

Servings: 8

Ingredients:

- 4 lb. chicken breasts, skinless and boneless
- 1 tbsp garlic powder
- 2 tbsp dried Italian herb mix
- 2 tbsp olive oil
- 1/4 cup chicken stock
- Pepper
- Salt

Directions:

1. Coat chicken with oil and season with dried herb, garlic powder, pepper, and salt. Place chicken into the Pressure Pot. Pour stock over the chicken. Seal pot with a lid and select manual and set timer for 12 minutes.

2. Once done, allow to release pressure naturally for 5 minutes then release remaining using quick release. Remove lid. Shred chicken using a fork and serve.

Nutrition:

Calories 502; Fat 20.8 g; Carbohydrates 7.8 g; Protein 66.8 g

Lightning Source UK Ltd.
Milton Keynes UK
UKHW020757230621
386009UK00001B/50